# WARFARIN
### &
# YOU

## V.B. BLAKE

Disclaimer:

The material in this publication was sourced from various internet websites. It is intended for information purposes only and should not be used in place of consultation with a health care professional. The author, publisher, participating retailers/ pharmacies, vendors, and/or agencies are not responsible for errors, omissions, or inconsistencies with respect to the information contained in this book and does not accept liability whatsoever for reliance by the reader on the information contained herein. The author acknowledges the trademarked status and trademark owners of various products referenced in this work, which have been used without permission. The publication/use of these trademarks is not authorized, associated with, or sponsored by the trademark owners.

To my mother.

# INTRODUCTION

There is much valuable information available on a wide variety of internet websites that will educate you on every type of blood clot imaginable, what symptoms to look for, complications, and so on. It is not the intent of this small publication to educate you thoroughly on the medical terminology and aspects of blood clots, which is a subject best left to the professional and highly trained individuals. I hope this brief compilation of information will provide a general overview of blood clots with dietary suggestions that will guide anyone who is taking the life-changing drug Warfarin in making better nutritional choices.

# Table of Contents

# FOREWARD

I am blessed with extremely good health and other than breaking a bone here and there during my fifty-nine years on this planet, I've had nothing to complain about. A couple of years ago, while spending a few months in the hospital for hip problems, my breathing became an issue and the doctors discovered an eight-inch blood clot in my lungs. Fortunately, they were able to break up the clot and save my life. Had I suffered a pulmonary embolism while at home I would have died. I understand I had a thirty-minute window before the embolism took my life and seeing as the nearest hospital is two hours away the chances of my survival would have been slim to none.

Before that event, I never gave blood clots a consideration other than thinking of them as small circular globs of blood that may have the misfortune of clogging veins. There wasn't any pain or discomfort prior to or after the event and other than my shallow breathing I felt fine. I understand there are some people who have no warning that there might be a problem, who just close their eyes never to open them again. My entire perception of blood clots has changed since that time, as you can imagine.

My doctor told me I would be on Warfarin for the rest of my life. I was familiar with Warfarin having had to take it after previous hip surgeries to eliminate the possibility of clotting, but I never thought my blood would actually cause a life long problem. I don't take any medication, as a rule, other than the odd dose of penicillin for mild infections and such, but now I faced a lifetime ingesting this drug daily.

When discharged from the hospital, I was given a couple of well-photocopied sheets of paper that briefly cautioned against consuming excessive amounts of Vitamin K while taking Warfarin. I didn't even know there was such a vitamin. That's when I knew I had to find as much information as I could about this drug that would be a part of my daily regime forever. After regaining my physical strength I brushed the dust off and fired up my computer to determine how I would live with the drug, Warfarin.

There was plenty of online information from a multitude of sources and after reading each website I had lots of academic knowledge but little practical knowledge. I thought about my mother who takes Warfarin and does not use a computer. She doesn't have access to these online information sources and has to rely on other means for data. Our local pharmacy provides a monograph for every new drug prescribed which highlights various side effects, interaction cautions, and so on, which is an excellent information resource.

During my internet exploration exercises I became aware that food can have a negative interaction on Warfarin, for example, eating leafy green vegetables such as spinach and romaine lettuce was a repeated concern. I'm a huge fan of Caesar, tossed, and spinach salads and wondered if I had to give them up altogether and what else was I eating that could potentially cause a problem? It would be stupid of me to spend the time and money to take a daily dose of Warfarin for the rest of my days if I was putting my life in jeopardy by countering the healing effects by eating the wrong foods. I knew I had to discover just which foods would hinder or help my new lifestyle.

I continued to search and soon found myself tangled within a sea of information written in medical terminology that made me dizzy. I couldn't find one little compact source written in layman's English that would give me an overview of information, a jumping off place, if you will. I didn't need to know all the medical words I just needed to understand what was going on in my body and what I could eat. Undaunted, I continued to compile information that helped me plan my new life living with Warfarin. When I had an understanding of my body functioning with Warfarin and an idea of what changes to make in my lifestyle and diet, I considered how this compilation might be able to help others in a similar situation.

I hope that you will find some benefit in this little guide and make choices that will make your journey with Warfarin a long and uneventful one.

# News Flash

As this publication was heading to the printer, the *New England Journal of Medicine* published their newest research on a study for an effective and safer treatment for patients coping with deep-vein thrombosis (DVT).

*Rivaroxaban* (Xarelto) is a new anti-clotting pill that the study has found to be safe and effective, although it costs more than regular drugs. The current standard of care typically involves treatment with relatively well-known anti-coagulant medications, such as the oral medication Warfarin (Coumadin) and/or the injected medication Heparin. For some patients the drug can have adverse effects and interact negatively with other medications. When taking Warfarin the potential also exists for the possibility of severe and life-threatening bleeding which is the reason intense and continuous monitoring is necessary. *Rivaroxiban* therapy is much easier for both the patient and physician since it does not require blood testing to adjust the dose.

In March 2009, the U.S. Food and Drug Administration advisory panel recommended the drug be approved, but agency review is ongoing pending further study.

SOURCES: American Society of Hematology, news release, Dec. 4, 2010; *New England Journal of Medicine*, Dec. 4, 2010, et. al.

# 1 WHAT IS A BLOOD CLOT?

Our bodies create blood clots as a normal response to blood vessel damage. Blood clots are semi-solid masses of sticky blood cells that form to seal the leak and stop the bleeding. Clots that block the arteries (*thrombi*) and prevent flow of blood and oxygen to an organ can lead to areas of tissue damage, also called *infarcts*. When blood clots break away (*embolism*) from the area that they're meant to protect, they can endanger other organs.

Clots that block blood flow are the main culprits in most heart attacks and strokes. They can also damage other organs as follows:

When a blood clot (*thrombus*) forms in one or more arteries that supply blood to the heart, it blocks the blood flow to a part of the heart muscle, reducing or completely cutting off the oxygen supply to the cells in that area. As a result, the part of the heart muscle that is deprived of oxygen dies, and a heart attack may occur.

Clots that block the flow of oxygen to the brain are the primary cause of strokes.

Clots that form in the eye may cause sudden blindness.

Presence of an obstructing blood clot (*thrombus*) is referred to as *thrombosis*. Thrombosis in a vein is almost always associated with *phlebitis* (an inflammation of a vein).

# Thrombophlebitis

*Thrombophlebitis* is an inflammation of a vein in the area where a blood clot has formed. Thrombophlebitis is classified as either superficial or deep. In other words, thrombosis can affect either superficial (surface) or deep (below the surface) veins causing thrombophlebitis.

# Superficial Thrombophlebitis

*Superficial thrombophlebitis* occurs when a blood clot affects veins near the skin surface, or superficial veins. A variety of things can cause inflammation of a superficial vein. One common cause is due to trauma or injury, for example, from solutions or medications given *intravenously* (into a vein) in hospitals. Piercing the vein to give the solution or medication can cause irritation. Any blow to a vein (such as an injury from a car accident) will trigger inflammation in the area, leading to pain, discomfort, redness, and swelling. During this process, there's an increased flow of blood to the injured area, and a blood clot often forms in the inflamed or injured area of the vein. Superficial thrombophlebitis is an uncomfortable condition but rarely causes serious problems.

Sometimes, thrombophlebitis is caused by a bacterial infection in the vein. The usual culprit is a bacteria called *Staphylococcus*, commonly found on the skin.

In certain cases, thrombophlebitis develops without an obvious reason. It may develop in the leg veins of pregnant women, in people with varicose veins, and in some people with cancer in the abdomen (particularly the pancreas). Women over the age of 35 years who smoke and take oral contraceptives (birth control pills) are at a higher risk of developing blood clots.

## Deep venous thrombosis (DVT)

*Deep venous thrombosis* (DVT) occurs when a blood clot affects deeper, larger veins, such as those in the lower legs and thighs. DVT is more worrisome than superficial thrombophlebitis. These clots can break away (clots that break away from a blood vessel are called *emboli*) and cause a pulmonary embolism if they travel to the lung. DVT is more common for people over 40 years of age.

DVT occurs when blood clots form in the deep veins of the legs or pelvis, and is often caused by:

- prolonged sitting or bed rest

- surgery or trauma (especially hip surgery, gynecological surgery, heart surgery)

- medications such as estrogen, and birth control pills with higher levels of estrogen

- injury to the leg or immobilization (such as casting after a broken bone).

Certain inherited conditions can make DVT more likely to occur. Blood flow in the veins depends on contraction of surrounding muscles, and with inactivity, such as extended bed rest, the blood starts to collect and blood clots can easily form.

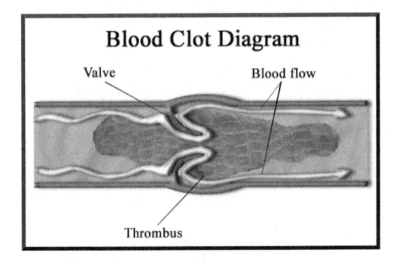

# Blood Clot Diagram

Valve

Blood flow

Thrombus

# 2 WHAT CAUSES BLOOD CLOTS?

Through media sources, we are increasingly aware of people in their 40s dropping dead from blood clots, and the numbers of heart attacks and stroke victims seems to be increasing as well. There doesn't seem to be any warning in most cases so what actually causes clots and is there anything we can actively do to prevent their forming?

## Trauma

Trauma can cause clots. We've all had a bruise at one time or another, usually caused by hitting parts of our bodies against immoveable objects. A bruise is simply a mark on our skin caused by blood that has been trapped under the surface because of the bump. The injury crushes small blood vessels that break open and leak blood under the skin. After a few days or so, the injury repairs itself and the bruise disappears. An injury that damages a blood vessel may develop a blood clot that will seal the leak otherwise we would bleed to death. While clots are necessary to stop bleeding and to help us heal, normally when they've done their jobs our body automatically dissolves them. It's when the clots persist that they cause problems.

A blood clot can be likened to a blob of jelly and are more commonly found in veins rather than arteries. To a non-professional, like myself, I never gave much thought to the difference between arteries and veins. As far as I was concerned, they both carried blood to and from my internal organs and that's the only consideration I gave to the subject. While I was in the hospital, and asking my usual abundance of questions, one nurse put it quite simply: veins carry blood to the organs and arteries carry blood away from the organs.

## Artery Blockage

When a clot blocks an artery, it is called *thrombi*. These *thrombi* prevent the flow of blood and oxygen to our organs and could cause tissue damage, called *infarcts*. Heart attacks may occur when a clot forms in one or more arteries that supply blood to the heart. These clots block the flow of blood to a part of the heart muscle that may reduce or cut off the oxygen supply to cells, and when a part of the heart muscle that is deprived of oxygen dies it may result in a heart attack. When a clot forms and blocks oxygen to the brain, it may cause a stroke. Clots that form in the eye may cause blindness.

## Cardiogenic embolisms

Cardiogenic embolisms are clots that have formed inside the heart and travel to the brain. A heart that has been damaged by a heart attack will not properly pump blood, which can cause blood clots that can travel to the brain. Artificial replacement heart valves are likely to form clots; however, by taking blood-thinning medication, it may prevent their formation. A stroke may occur in someone who has suffered a heart attack.

## Atrial fibrillation

Atrial fibrillation is an irregular heartbeat (*arrhythmia*) that causes a rapid, quivering beat in the upper chamber of the heart (*atria*). As a result of the irregular pumping, some blood may remain in the heart chamber and form clots which can then travel to the brain, resulting in a stroke.

In about 15% of all *ischemic strokes* (strokes caused by blood clots lodging in the brain), blood clots may form in the heart as a result of the rhythm disorder known as *atrial fibrillation.* Emboli can also form at the site of artificial heart valves, after a heart attack, or as a result of heart valve disorder or heart failure.

## Pulmonary embolisms

Pulmonary embolisms occur when a blood clot in the veins breaks away and moves to the lungs where it could block the airways. A large clot results in increased difficulty in breathing, and even death.

## Atherosclerosis

Atherosclerosis is commonly known as hardening of the arteries. This is caused when, over time, the arterial walls slowly thicken, harden, and narrow until normal blood flow is reduced. If the walls tear a blood clot may form and completely block the already narrowed artery and shut off oxygen to part of the heart or brain.

## Oral Contraceptives

Oral contraceptives taken by women over 35 years of age, who smoke and have a history of previous blood clots, have an increased risk of blood clot formation.

## Hormone replacement therapy

Menopausal women using hormone replacement therapy, especially a combination of estrogen and progestin, are more likely to develop deep vein thrombosis, which can lead to a pulmonary embolism.

## Infection

Studies have shown some evidence that infection (e.g., urinary tract infection, respiratory infection) can increase the risk of blood clot formation, particularly deep vein thrombosis.

## Periods of inactivity

Long periods of inactivity may increase the risk for blood clots. Examples include long road trips by car, long air flights, and extensive bed rest due to illness or surgery.

Blood clotting problems and rare blood disorders also cause blood clots to form, but the cause of blood clots is not always known.

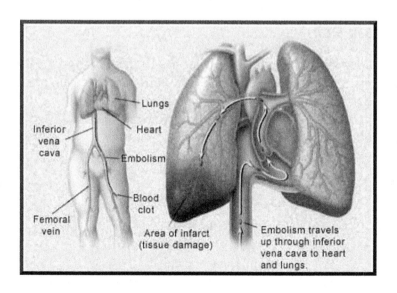

# 3 HOW DO I KNOW IF I HAVE BLOOD CLOTS?

## Leg Pain

It depends where the blood clot has formed. In most cases, it is the legs, especially the calf area, however, at least 30% of people with a clot will not have any symptoms. Those who do may have some of the following symptoms:

- a heavy feeling in the leg

- tenderness in the calf area

- swelling in the calf area

- warmth near the calf

# Heart Attack

Blood clots causing heart attacks may cause chest pain *(angina)* that usually starts in the centre of the chest and moves to the jaw, the back, the left arm, or occasionally, the right arm. Less commonly, the pain may be felt in the abdomen. Heart attack pain is usually severe but not always. You may have some of the following symptoms:

- abdominal pain

- a feeling of impending doom

- tightness or a pounding in the chest

- increased heart speed and irregular beat

- shortness of breath

- difficulty breathing

- nausea or vomiting

- fainting or collapse

Some people have *silent heart attacks* without any symptoms. Women may experience slightly different symptoms than men, and are more likely to experience nausea and less likely to sweat and the chest pain may not be felt as distinctly as in men. The most common places for women's chest pain to spread to are the neck, jaw, or back.

# Stroke

Blood clots causing a stroke usually result in symptoms occurring on the opposite side of the body from where they form in the brain. You may have some of the following symptoms:

- loss of feeling on one side of the face, arm or leg, or blindness

- problems with speech

- unable to speak or understand spoken words

- confusion

- severe headache

- sudden loss of coordination or balance

- double vision

- abnormal eye movements

- a gray shading or fogging within the field of vision

Signs of stroke should not be ignored, however brief or seemingly insignificant. Even if symptoms only last a few minutes and then vanish completely, it is important to seek medical attention right away.

# Deep Vein Thrombosis

Deep vein thrombosis is an inflammation of a superficial vein. Some medical sources report DVT is occurring at a high incidence rate, even going so far as to call if epidemic. When blood clots form in the deep veins of the legs or pelvis, you may have some of these symptoms:

- swelling
- pain or tenderness over a vein
- sharp pain when flexing the foot
- redness
- warm sensation over the affected area
- aching tightness in the calf, especially when walking
- widening of the surface leg veins

# Pulmonary Embolism

Pulmonary embolism is a blood clot that has formed in the deeper, larger veins, usually in the legs, abdomen, and pelvis, that has broken away. Known as a travelling blood clot, or *embolus*, it can travel and lodge in the lung. You may have some of the following symptoms:

- breathlessness
- chest pain
- bloody sputum

# 4 HOW ARE BLOOD CLOTS DIAGNOSED?

**Superficial thrombophlebitis** is usually diagnosed according to your symptoms. A doctor will take your medical history by asking about your symptoms and conducting a physical examination.

In the case of **thrombophlebitis**, an ultrasound of the suspected veins may be done to confirm the diagnosis. Since the leg pain associated with DVT is very similar to muscle pain, your doctor might look for signs of swelling and enlargement of the calf due to swollen leg veins.

A diagnosis of **DVT** is usually confirmed with a *compression ultrasound*. Compression ultrasound detects differences in echoes or sounds made by flowing blood, and can easily detect the presence of blood clots in deep veins.

# 5 HOW ARE BLOOD CLOTS TREATED?

Medications are usually used to stop progression of DVT and prevent the blood clot from worsening, breaking away, and moving to the lungs. Blood-thinning medications such as Warfarin or Heparin are usually recommended. These medications may be continued for several months after a blood clot has been diagnosed. Most people do not require admission to a hospital to treat DVT, and those with DVT can usually return to normal activities within two to three weeks.

For some people, long-term treatment with Warfarin (an anticoagulant) may be necessary to prevent new blood clots from forming and painkillers may be used to reduce the pain. Your doctor may also recommend that you wear an elastic support stocking on your leg to prevent DVT.

To relieve mild inflammation and discomfort, the affected area should be elevated and warm moist packs applied for 15 to 20 minutes at a time throughout the day.

For people with *superficial thrombophlebitis*, activities such as walking are recommended. If the inflammation and symptoms last longer than a day or two, or if symptoms become worse, see a doctor as soon as possible.

In cases where the *thrombophlebitis* is due to an infection, treatment with antibiotics often takes care of the problem. In rare cases, when the antibiotics aren't enough to control the infection, surgical removal of the inflamed portion of the vein may be required.

Prevention of blood clots is the best way to deal with the problems of heart disease and stroke. It is important to reduce or quit smoking and to control high blood pressure. High cholesterol levels also present a risk for blood clots and may be checked by your doctor. A healthy diet and regular exercise also help to reduce the risk of heart attack and stroke.

Anticoagulants like Warfarin block the action of Vitamin K. In turn, Vitamin K blocks the action of anticoagulants. This is why people taking Wafarin have to limit how much Vitamin K they get in their diet.

# 6 CAN I TRAVEL?

To help prevent DVT, avoid long periods of immobility such as those during long car trips or airplane flights; try to walk around and stretch for a few minutes every hour or so. Elevate your legs above your heart level if possible, and if you have a history of blood clots, wear support stockings or socks.

Wear a medical alert tag or carry an ID card stating that you take Warfarin.

# 7 WHAT IS WARFARIN?

Warfarin is also known under the brand names Coumadin, Jantoven, Marevan, and Waran. Warfarin belongs to the class of medications called anticoagulants and is prescribed to people with an increased tendency for *thrombosis* or, to those who have experienced blood clots, to prevent further occurrences. Frequently, it is referred to as a blood thinner, although it does not actually thin the blood. Warfarin does not dissolve blood clots; rather, it helps to prevent blood clots from forming or getting larger.

It works by partially blocking the reuse of Vitamin K in your liver, which is needed to make clotting factors that help the blood to clot and prevent bleeding. Vitamin K is found naturally in foods such as leafy, green vegetables, and some vegetable oils. Sudden changes in the amount of Vitamin K you consume can affect how Warfarin works.

Warfarin is the most widely prescribed anticoagulant drug in North America but despite its effectiveness, treatment with Warfarin has several shortcomings. Many commonly used medications interact with Warfarin, as do some foods, which may enhance or reduce its anticoagulation effect. It is, therefore, extremely important that its activity is monitored by frequent blood testing to determine the degree of anticoagulation.

Blood clots in the circulation are dangerous because they can cause medical problems such as heart attacks, stroke, and pulmonary embolism. Warfarin helps to reduce blood clotting within 24 hours of taking the medication while the full effect may take 72 to 96 hours to occur.

Do not stop taking this medication without consulting your doctor. Do not give this medication to anyone else, even if they have the same symptoms as you do. It can be harmful for people to take this medication if their doctor has not prescribed it.

The dose of Warfarin is individualized by your doctor according to blood clotting time as determined by laboratory tests, called an INR (*international normalized ratio*), performed at regular intervals. It is very important to keep your lab appointments as there is a narrow range between too much and too little of the medication. Too much medication may cause you to bleed more and too little medication may let a harmful clot form.

Different circumstances in your life (e.g., eating certain foods or using certain medications) can cause Warfarin to work more or less effectively. It is very important that you take Warfarin exactly as prescribed by your doctor. If you miss a dose of Warfarin, take the missed dose as soon as possible and continue with your regular schedule. If it is almost time for your next dose, skip the missed dose and continue with your regular dosing schedule. **Do not take a double dose to make up for a missed one.** If you are not sure what to do after missing a dose, contact your doctor or pharmacist for advice.

Store this medication at room temperature, protect it from light and moisture, and keep it out of the reach of children.

While you are taking Warfarin, your lifestyle choices may change as follows:

- do not make drastic changes in your diet, such as eating large amounts of green, leafy vegetables

- do not attempt to change your weight by dieting without first checking with your doctor

- do not participate in any activity or sport that may result in serious injury

- avoid drinking alcohol

- avoid cutting yourself

Before you start Warfarin treatment, tell your doctor about all other diseases you have and all the medicines, including over the counter drugs, herbs, herbal teas, vitamins, alternative medicines and special diets you are on. Many medications such as aspirin, acetaminophen (Tylenol) and ibuprofen (Advil, Motrin), and herbs, such as gingko, danshen and devil's claw increase the effect of Warfarin. Some sedatives, coenzyme Q, and ginseng decrease the effect of Warfarin.

More than 2 million Americans experience a DVT each year. These leg clots can migrate to the lungs to form potentially deadly pulmonary embolisms.

# 8 IS WARFARIN A BLOOD THINNER?

While many people are prescribed Warfarin as a blood thinner to prevent the formation of clots, it does not actually thin the blood. Warfarin belongs to the class of medications called *anticoagulants.* It has a narrow therapeutic margin, which means that any change in the amount of Warfarin in your bloodstream may change the way the drug affects you. For example, too much Warfarin may cause excessive bleeding, while too little could affect the drug's ability to prevent clots, and this could lead to serious health effects, such as a heart attack or stroke.

# 9 WHAT IS COUMADIN?

Coumadin is a brand name, as are Jantoven, Marevan, and Waran, for the drug Warfarin.

You may need to stop taking Warfarin for a short time if you need antibiotics, surgery, dental work, a spinal tap, or spinal anesthesia (epidural).

# 10 ARE THERE ANY SIDE EFFECTS?

The common side effect of Warfarin is bleeding although the risk of severe bleeding is small. The risk of bleeding is increased if the INR (*international normalized ratio)* is out of range; too little medication may result in blood clots forming or too much medication may result in bleeding.

Some symptoms, which may occur, are:

- nausea, vomiting, loss of appetite, stomach/abdominal bloating or cramps

- coughing up blood

- excessive bruising

- bleeding from the nose or gums

- blood in urine or stool

Symptoms of a serious allergic reaction may include:

- rash

- itching

- swelling

- severe dizziness

- trouble breathing

If any of these effects persist or worsen, notify your doctor or pharmacist immediately.

Although a pulmonary embolism can arise from anywhere in the body, most commonly it arises from the calf veins.

# 11 ARE THERE ANY ADVERSE REACTIONS TO OTHER DRUGS

Many prescription and over-the-counter drug products are known to interact with Warfarin. Some examples of drug classes are:

- antibiotics

- non-steroidal anti-inflammatory agents (Acetylsalicylic acid [ASA], celecoxib)

- acetaminophen

- antidepressants

- stomach ulcer/acid reducing agents

- lipid lowering agents

- antifungal agents

It is important that your doctor is aware of all the prescription, over-the-counter, and herbal medications you are taking since caffeine, alcohol, nicotine, or illegal drugs can affect the effectiveness of Warfarin. Over-the-counter anti-inflammatory medications, such as aspirin or ibuprofen, may increase the risk of bleeding. You can usually take acetaminophen (Tylenol®), but if taken more than once a day and for longer than a week, you should tell your doctor.

**Purple Toes Syndrome** is a complication of Warfarin treatment, which results in dark, purplish, or mottled colour of toes that usually happens 3-10 weeks, or later, after treatment begins.

The syndrome consists of the following major features:

- an increase and decrease of the colour

- pain and tenderness of the toes

- purple colour under and at the sides of the toes that turns white when moderate pressure is applies and fades when the legs are raised

# Alcohol

Drinking 1-2 glasses of wine or 1-2 beers per day usually does not influence the INR and will not increase the risk for bleeding. However, drinking a large amount of alcohol can affect the way Warfarin works and increase your risk for bleeding.

## Natural Herbs

Warfarin also interacts with many herbs, for example:

- ginger, which is taken for nausea and poor digestion

- garlic, used to help lower high cholesterol levels, high triglycerides, and high blood pressure, when used as a supplement, not in the diet or for medicinal purposes

- ginseng, taken to help with fatigue and weakness

- ginkgo (a.k.a. Ginkgo Biloba), used to increase brain blood flow, prevent dementia, and improve memory, may all increase bleeding and bruising in people taking Warfarin, similar effects have been reported with borage (starflower) oil or fish oils

- St. John's Wort, sometimes recommended to help with mild to moderate depression, interacts with Warfarin causing a reduced anticoagulant effect

## NSAIDs

It is recommended that anyone taking non-steroidal anti-inflammatory agents (NSAIDs) such as ASA or ibuprofen should be closely monitored to ensure that no change in anticoagulation dosage is required. NSAIDs can cause stomach ulcers or bleeding.

## Pregnancy

Warfarin should not be used during pregnancy.

## Breast-feeding

It is not known if Warfarin passes into human breast milk, however, if you are a breast-feeding mother and are taking this medication it may affect your baby. Talk to your doctor about whether you should continue breast-feeding.

## Children

The safety and effectiveness of this medication for children under 18 years of age have not been established. However, the use of Warfarin by children is necessary in certain situations and any concerns you may have should be discussed with your physician.

While taking Warfarin, potential exists for the development of severe and life-threatening bleeding. Intense and continuous monitoring is essential..

# 12 WHY DO I NEED REGULAR BLOOD TESTS?

Regular blood tests are important. A blood test called an INR is required to determine how much Warfarin you need. Because many factors can influence how your body responds to Warfarin, you will need to have regular blood tests as long as you are taking it. Your doctor will determine the range of INR that is right for you and decide how frequently it should be checked. Normally, INR is checked at least once a month, but more frequent testing may be appropriate in some situations. Try to have your test performed in the morning on a weekday so your doctor can adjust your dose if necessary.

# 13 WHEN SHOULD I CONTACT MY PHYSICIAN?

The following side effects have been reported by at least 1% of people taking this medication. Many of these side effects can be managed, and some may go away on their own over time. Contact your doctor if you experience these side effects and they are severe or bothersome. Your pharmacist may be able to advise you on managing side effects.

- diarrhea

- intolerance to cold

- loss of appetite

- nausea or vomiting

- stomach cramps or pain

Although most of the side effects listed below don't happen very often they could lead to serious problems if you do not check with your doctor or seek medical attention. Check with your doctor as soon as possible if any of the following side effects occur:

- bleeding from cuts that need a long time to stop

- bleeding gums

- headaches, dizziness, or weakness

- heavier than normal menstrual bleeding

- nosebleeds

- numbness or tingling of hands, feet, or face

- pain, swelling, or discomfort

- paralysis

- pink or brown urine

- sudden shortness of breath

- unexplained bruising

- unusual pain or swelling

Stop taking the medication and seek immediate medical attention if *any* of the following occur:

- fainting

- signs of a serious allergic reaction (i.e., swelling of face or throat, hives, or difficulty breathing)

- signs of bleeding (dark, tarry stools, bleeding in eye, blood in stools, blood in vomit or vomit that looks like coffee grounds, blood in urine, coughing up blood)

- signs of liver damage (i.e., yellowing of skin or eyes, dark urine, light-coloured stools)

Some people may experience side effects other than those listed. Check with your doctor if you notice any symptom that worries you while you are taking this medication.

Inform your doctor if you develop side effects, miss a dose; change your diet, medications, herbs or supplements; become ill, have a surgical or dental procedure planned, or plan to travel. If you become pregnant.

If you get sick while on Warfarin the illness may affect your body's response to Warfarin.

If you develop a viral or bacterial infection, an episode of congestive heart failure, or nausea, vomiting or diarrhea lasting more than 24 hours.

If you plan to travel, carry identification explaining the reason you are taking Warfarin, the target range for INR, and current dosage. Carry the Warfarin record sheet (ask your doctor for a copy) and make sure you have enough Warfarin to last through your trip. Carry your medications with you at all times - do not put medications in checked baggage and try to maintain your usual diet.

If you have to see other health care providers, i.e., specialists, emergency room physicians, dentists, pharmacists, etc., tell them that you are taking Warfarin.

If you do not have a regular doctor and have been started on Warfarin in hospital, it is critical that you immediately find a regular doctor to monitor your proper Warfarin dosage. If you cannot find a regular doctor, contact a hospital doctor for assistance.

The primary symptoms associated with vitamin K deficiencies are osteoporosis and prolonged bleeding times. Other symptoms that occur frequently in conjunction with osteoporosis and prolonged bleeding times in connective tissue disorders are mitral valve prolapse, scoliosis and hypermobility.

# 14 ISN'T WARFARIN USED IN PESTICIDES?

The use of Warfarin as pesticide has declined because many rat populations have developed resistance to it and poisons of considerably greater potency are now available.

If you miss a dose, take the missed dose as soon as you remember, and call your doctor as soon as possible. Do not take two doses at the same time to make up a missed dose.

# 15 WHO SHOULDN'T TAKE WARFARIN?

Warfarin should not be taken by anyone who:

- is allergic to Warfarin or to any of the ingredients of the medication

- is pregnant

- is undergoing certain types of anaesthesia

- does not have access to an adequate lab facility to get regular blood tests done

- has a high risk of abortion, eclampsia, and preeclampsia (complications of pregnancy often associated with sudden onset of very high blood pressure)

- has bleeding tendencies associated with active ulcers or overt bleeding of the stomach, genitourinary, or respiratory tracts, or bleeding associated with many other medical conditions

- has bleeding tendencies or blood disorders

- has malignant hypertension

- has recently had or is planning to have surgery of the central nervous system or the eye or surgery associated with trauma resulting in large open surfaces

- has senility, alcoholism, or psychosis, or other conditions where the person may not be able to cooperate with taking the medication and having the necessary lab tests on a regular basis.

The bacteria that synthesize Vitamin K thrive in an acidic digestive environment. Antacids, if taken in sufficient quantity, may cause a Vitamin K deficiency, as well as irritable bowel syndrome and various nutritional deficiencies, because they neutralize the hydrochloric acid in a person's stomach. Hydrochloric acid is needed to digest food and create the acidic environment in which the beneficial bacteria thrive.

# 16 SHOULD I TAKE NATURAL OR HERBAL PRODUCTS?

There are a number of natural health and food products that may affect Warfarin levels in different ways, for example, research has shown that the popular herbal product ginseng can reduce the effects of Warfarin, while taking ginkgo biloba may increase its effects. Both of these changes pose health risks because the effect of Warfarin on blood clotting must remain stable in your system to be safe and effective.

Over time researchers will no doubt discover new information about products that can alter the effects of Warfarin. To date, there is evidence that the following herbal, vitamin and mineral products may change levels of Warfarin in the bloodstream or may directly affect blood clotting on their own:

- chondroitin plus glucosamine

- coenzyme Q10 - also known as ubiquinone, ubidecarenone

- danshen

- devil's claw

- dong quai - also known as Danggui, Chinese Angelica

- feverfew

- fenugreek together with boldo

- fish oil supplements that contain eicosapentaenoic acid (EPA) and docosahexaenoic acid (DHA);

- ginkgo biloba

- ginseng (*Panax ginseng*) - also known as Asian ginseng, Chinese ginseng, Japanese ginseng, Korean ginseng

- American ginseng

- green tea

- horse chestnut

- Chinese Wolfberry, Di Gu Pi, Goji Berry, Gou Qi Zi

- papaya extract (containing papain)

- certain brands of *quilinggao* - also known as "essence of tortoise shell"

- St. John's Wort

- vitamin A

- vitamin K

- wintergreen (used on the skin)

- There is also evidence that the following food products may affect Warfarin levels:

- avocado

- cranberry juice

- flax (flaxseed)

- garlic

- ginger

- mango

- onions

- papaya

- seaweed (sushi wrap)

- soy protein products (including soymilk and tofu)

# 17 WHAT IS *COLEUS FORSKOLIN?*

Most people have never heard of *Coleus Forskolin* but it could be one of the super supplements that can help alleviate a variety of health problems. The coleus plant grows in India and surrounding countries and is sold as *coleus extract* or *coleus forskohlii* extract. Forskolin extract is believed by many alternative medical experts to cure almost every kind of disease known to man. While most of these supplements are exaggerated, there is some research to indicate that there are beneficial effects on health, if not quite as wonderful as advertised. Forskolin extract could be one of those that actually come close to living up to the hype.

As more and more people are turning to natural herbs and supplements they are finding that many of these do not work. One of the exceptions may be coleus forskolin extract. Its benefits for helping with reducing blood clot formations, depression, glaucoma, and heart disease, if true, can help thousands of people in their search for better health. Coleus plants and coleus extract don't seem to have any adverse effect so what is the harm in trying?

Coleus extract is thought to activate *adentyl cyclase*, which enhances cellular functioning. The coleus plant is thought to be a very effective weight loss supplement and has been shown in some research to actually increase the metabolism of fat. Some people have reported losing up to ten pounds within a few months of taking coleus forskolin extract.

One of the most important effects of coleus plants is that it is believed to aid in reducing the risk of blood clots. Blood clots in the circulatory system are known to affect and increase the prevalence of heart disease and stroke. Because coleus extract also decreases blood pressure it has an added benefit to the heart. Because these disorders are common and life threatening using coleus forskolii extract can serve as a life line to those suffering from high blood pressure.

Coleus plants and coleus forskolin extract are considered to have many other health benefits as well, for example, coleus forskolin can be used to fight depression. By aiding cellular health it is believed to increase the effectiveness or neurotransmitters in the brain. When these neurotransmitters perform more efficiently they seem to increase the level of serotonin, which is the cause of most mood disorders.

Coleus forskolii extract from coleus plants are used as a cancer preventative. Because coleus extract affects the body on a cellular level, it is thought that it may help the body better fight cancerous cells before they develop.

Another benefit related to coleus forskolin seems to have is on glaucoma. Glaucoma is a disease that affects the eyes. Increased pressure because of glaucoma can and often does result in blindness. There has been research indicating that coleus extract from coleus plants reduces ocular pressure when taken consistently. However, it has only been shown to be effective for short periods.

People who are taking Warfarin should consult their doctors before starting vitamin, nutritional, or herbal therapies.

> Antibiotics can cause bleeding problems from Vitamin K deficiencies. Antibiotics destroy not only harmful digestive tract bacteria, but also the beneficial intestinal bacteria that is needed to create Vitamin K. In order to replace the beneficial intestinal bacteria after a course of antibiotics it is often recommended to eat yogurt with active cultures or have to take probiotic supplements containing acidophilus. Replacing beneficial bacteria after antibiotics is standard conventional medical advice in many European countries, but does not seem to be common medical advice in the United States.

# 18 WHAT ARE OTHER IMPORTANT SAFETY CONSIDERATIONS?

Keep your health professional up to date about the medications and natural health products you use, including vitamins, minerals and herbal products. Health Canada recommends the following:

- take the prescribed dose of Warfarin at the same time each day

- have your blood tested regularly for its clotting time

- talk to your health professional before you start taking any new drug and/or natural health products because your dose of Warfarin may have to be adjusted

- if you are already taking drug and/or natural health products and Warfarin, do not change your routine unless you have discussed it with your health professional

- ask your health professional about foods that may change the effects of Warfarin or have a direct effect on blood clotting

- if you eat or drink food products that can change the effects of Warfarin, be sure to keep your intake levels consistent from day to day

- if you have any unusual bruising or bleeding, contact your health care professional for advice right away

- do not start or stop any new medications, vitamins, herbs or supplements without telling your doctor

- avoid heavy or "binge" alcohol consumption. - moderate, consistent alcohol intake does not influence Warfarin therapy

## Other precautions:

- avoid any activity or sport that may result in a serious fall or other injury

- use a soft toothbrush, and brush and floss gently to prevent bleeding from the gums

- be careful when using razors

- use an electric razor if possible

- consider carrying a wallet card that explains that you are taking Warfarin.

Soybean, canola and vegetable oils are high in Vitamin K, however that doesn't mean one should eliminate these oils from diets. Exposure of oils to sunlight or fluorescent light destroys approximately 85% of the Vitamin K. You must expose them to sunlight or fluorescent light for at least 48 hours. When exposing the oils to sunlight, it is not necessary to expose the oil to open air. A transparent container in the sun will do the trick.

# 19 WHAT IS VITAMIN K?

Vitamin K is a fat-soluble vitamin that is needed for blood clotting. The body stores very little of this vitamin, which is rapidly depleted without regular dietary intake. If different amounts of Vitamin K (high one day and low the next day) are ingested, it will be more difficult to regulate clotting time. Food with high levels of Vitamin K are known to decrease the effects of Warfarin, such as liver, broccoli, brussels sprouts, and green leafy vegetables (e.g., spinach, Swiss chard, coriander, collards and cabbage). If you take Warfarin you should avoid sudden changes in your daily intake of these foods.

There have also been reports about a possible interaction between Warfarin and cranberry, so patients taking Warfarin have been advised to limit or avoid drinking cranberry juice.

# Vitamin K Deficiency

Deficiency can result in impaired blood clotting which is usually discovered by regular blood tests. Some symptoms may include:

- easy bruising and bleeding

- nosebleeds

- bleeding gums

- blood in the urine

- blood in the stool

- tarry black stools

- extremely heavy menstrual bleeding

Vitamin K deficiency is relatively uncommon in healthy adults, however, people at risk include those taking vitamin K antagonist anticoagulant drugs and individuals with significant liver damage or disease. Additionally, individuals with disorders of fat malabsorption may be at increased risk of vitamin K deficiency.

In infants, vitamin K deficiency may result in life-threatening bleeding within the skull (*intracranial hemorrhage*). Newborn babies who are exclusively breast-fed are at increased risk of vitamin K deficiency because human milk is relatively low in vitamin K compared to formula.

## How much Vitamin K do I need daily?

I've discovered resources where the daily intake of Vitamin K for women 19-70+ years of age is 90 micrograms (mcg) per day 120 mcg per day for men ages 19 to 70+ years, and others that indicate 65 mcg for women and 80 mcg for men. It isn't necessary to avoid foods with Vitamin K just keep your consumption fairly consistent rather than consuming a lot one day and very little the next.

## How do I know I'm getting enough Vitamin K in my daily diet?

The list below of some common foods and beverages, portion size, and the amount of Vitamin K per portion can help you monitor the amount of Vitamin K in your diet.

The amount of Vitamin K may vary depending on how the food is packaged and prepared, portion size, and other factors.

# 20 SHOULD I CHANGE MY DIET?

A diet that is low in saturated fats, high in fibre and contains plenty of fruit and vegetables helps to reduce the risk of *atherosclerosis*, a form of heart disease, in which fatty deposits build up in the linings of the blood vessels. This can lead to *thrombosis*, which occurs when one of the fatty plaques narrow a blood vessel and a blood clot or *thrombus*, forms, blocking the flow of blood.

Cut down on food high in saturated fat, such as dairy products, as well as foods that have a high salt content (which can raise blood pressure), such as yeast extract, bacon or sausages.

The risk of thrombosis increases with age, while other factors known to make it more likely include obesity.

Not all fats are bad for you. Some polyunsaturated fats contain omega-3 fatty acids, which make blood platelets less *sticky* to help to prevent blood clots. They are found in oily fish such as mackerel, herring and trout. Try to eat a meal including one of these fish two or three times a week.

Raw onion is thought to guard against the harmful effects of fatty foods by increasing the rate at which blood clots are broken down.

Fresh garlic is also thought to reduce the risk of blood clots, however, you would have to eat ten or more cloves a day for a significant effect.

> *"It is important for the production of many nutrients that we keep our "friendly" colon bacteria active and doing their job; to aid this process we should minimize our use of oral antibiotics, avoid excess sugars and processed foods, and occasionally evaluate and treat any abnormal organisms interfering in our colon, such as yeasts or parasites."*
>
> *"Yogurt, kefir, and acidophilus milk may help to increase the functioning of the intestinal bacterial flora and therefore contribute to vitamin K production."*
>
> *from "Vitamin K", by Elson M. Haas M.D.*

# 21 WHAT FOODS SHOULD I INCLUDE IN MY DIET?

Taking Warfarin won't necessarily require an overhaul of your favourite food choices so there is no need to discontinue enjoying dark leafy greens and cranberries on a regular basis. Eat what you want but keep your portions consistent and make sure your INR stays in range with the correct dose.

A diet containing too much meat increases the risk of *thrombosis,* or blood clotting, while a diet rich in fruit and vegetables reduces the risk of *thrombosis* that often occurs in the deep veins in the legs. Eating fish once or more often a week reduces the risk of *thrombosis* by between 30 and 45 percent.

The following list is by no means complete, but it will give you an overview of Vitamin K enriched foods.

# Vitamin K Foods

|  | *Portion* | *Micrograms* |
|---|---|---|

## GRAIN PRODUCTS

|  | Portion | Micrograms |
|---|---|---|
| Bagel, plain, | 4" | 1.0 |
| Bread, assorted types | 1 slice | 0.8 |
| Cereal | ½ cup | 2.1 |
| Flour, all types | 1 cup | 0.4 |
| Noodles, egg, spinach | 1 cup | 161.8 |
| Oatmeal | 1 cup | 7.5 |
| Pie crust, cookie-type, prepared from recipe, graham cracker, baked | 1 shell | 59.0 |
| Rice, white | 1 cup | 0.0 |
| Spaghetti, cooked | 1 cup | 0.0 |

## DAIRY PRODUCTS/EGGS

|  | Portion | Micrograms |
|---|---|---|
| Butter | 1 tbsp | 1.0 |
| Cheddar cheese | 1 oz. | 0.8 |
| Eggs, cooked | 1 large | 2.6 |
| Sour Cream, cultured | 1 tbsp | 0.1 |
| Yogurt, plain, whole milk | 8 oz. | 0.5 |
| Ice cream, vanilla | ½ cup | 0.2 |

# FRUITS

| | | |
|---|---|---|
| Apple | 1 | 3.0 |
| Banana | 1 | 0.6 |
| Blackberries, raw | 1 cup | 28.5 |
| Blueberries, raw | 1 cup | 28.0 |
| Blueberries, frozen, sweetened | 1 cup | 40.7 |
| Blueberry pie | 1 piece | 12.3 |
| Cantaloupe | 1/8 melon | 1.7 |
| Grapes, red or green | 10 grapes | 7.3 |
| Grapefruit | ½ | 0.0 |
| Kiwi fruit, fresh, raw | 1 medium | 30.6 |
| Lemon | 1 | 0.0 |
| Nuts, pine nuts, pignolia, dried | 1 oz | 15.3 |
| Nuts, chestnuts, European, roast | 1 cup | 11.2 |
| Orange | 1 | 0.0 |
| Peach | 1 | 2.5 |
| Pears, Asian, raw | 1 | 12.4 |
| Plums, dried (prunes), stewed | 1 cup | 64.7 |

| Plums, canned, purple, heavy syrup pack, solids and liquids | 1 cup | 11.1 |
|---|---|---|
| Raspberries, frozen, red, sweetened | 1 cup | 16.3 |
| Rhubarb, frozen, with sugar | 1 cup | 71.0 |

## MEAT

| Beef | 3 oz. | 1.9 |
|---|---|---|
| Chicken | 1 cup | 4.3 |
| Ham | 2 slices | 0.0 |
| Salmon | 3 oz. | 0.3 |
| Pork | 3 oz. | 0.0 |
| Shrimp | 3 oz. | 0.0 |
| Tuna, light, canned in oil | 3 oz. | 37.4 |
| Tuna, light, canned in water | 3 oz. | 0.2 |
| Turkey meat only, roasted | 1 cup | 5.2 |
| Turkey patties, breaded, battered, fried | 1 patty | 13.4 |

## FATS AND DRESSINGS

| Margarine | 1 tbsp | 14.5 |
|---|---|---|
| Margarine-butter blend, 60% corn oil margarine and 40% butter | 1 tbsp | 14.7 |

| | | |
|---|---|---|
| Margarine, vegetable oil spread, 60% fat, stick | 1 tbsp | 14.5 |
| Margarine, regular, tub, composite, 80% fat, with salt | 1 tbsp | 13.2 |
| Margarine, regular, unspecified oils, w/salt added | 1 tbsp | 13.1 |
| Mayonnaise | 1 tbsp | 5.8 |

## Oils

| | | |
|---|---|---|
| Soybean | 1 tbsp | 3.4 |
| Olive | 1 tbsp | 8.1 |
| Corn | 1 tbsp | 0.3 |
| Peanut | 1 tbsp | 0.1 |
| Safflower | 1 tbsp | 1.0 |
| Sesame | 1 tbsp | 1.8 |
| Sunflower | 1 tbsp | 0.7 |

## VEGETABLES

| | | |
|---|---|---|
| Artichokes, (globe or french) | 1 cup | 24.9 |
| Asparagus, frozen, cooked | 1 cup | 144.0 |
| Asparagus, cooked | 4 spears | 30.4 |
| Avocado | 1 oz. | 6.0 |
| Beans, green | 1 cup | 20.0 |

| | | |
|---|---|---|
| Beans, snap, yellow, cooked | 1 cup | 20.0 |
| Beans, snap, green, cooked | 1 cup | 20.0 |
| Broccoli, cooked | 1 cup | 220.1 |
| Broccoli, raw | 1 spear | 31.5 |
| Brussels sprouts, cooked | 1 cup | 218.9 |
| Cabbage, raw | 1 cup | 53.2 |
| Cabbage, chinese (pak-choi), cooked, boiled, drained | 1 cup | 57.8 |
| Cabbage, savoy, raw | 1 cup | 48.2 |
| Cabbage, red, raw | 1 cup | 26.7 |
| Carrots | 1 cup | 21.4 |
| Carrots, frozen | 1 cup | 19.9 |
| Carrots, canned, regular pack | 1 cup | 14.3 |
| Carrot juice, canned | 1 cup | 36.6 |
| Cauliflower, boiled | 1 cup | 17.1 |
| Cauliflower, frozen, | 1 cup | 21.4 |
| Celery | 1 cup | 56.7 |
| Celery, raw | 1 stalk | 11.7 |
| Celery, cooked | 1 stalk | 14.2 |
| Coleslaw, fast foods | 3/4 cup | 56.4 |
| Collard greens | 1 cup | 1059.4 |

| | | |
|---|---|---|
| Corn | 1 cup | 0.5 |
| Cowpeas (blackeyes), immature seeds, frozen, boiled | 1 cup | 62.6 |
| Cucumber, peel removed | 1 cup | 8.6 |
| Cucumber, with peel, raw | 1 large | 49.4 |
| Dandelion greens, cooked, | 1 cup | 203.6 |
| Eggplant, cooked | 1 cup | 2.9 |
| Endive, raw | 1 cup | 115.5 |
| Kale, frozen, cooked, no salt | 1 cup | 1146.6 |
| Kale, cooked, no salt | 1 cup | 1062.1 |
| Lettuce, romaine or green leaf | 1 cup | 97.2 |
| Lettuce, iceberg, raw | 1 cup | 13.3 |
| Lettuce, Boston and bibb, raw | 1 head | 166.7 |
| Mung beans, mature seeds, sprouted, raw | 1 cup | 34.3 |
| Mushrooms | 1 cup | 0.2 |
| Mustard greens, cooked | 1 cup | 419.3 |
| Okra, frozen, cooked | 1 cup | 88.0 |
| Okra, cooked, boiled | 1 cup | 64.0 |
| Parsley | 10 sprigs | 164.0 |
| Peas, cooked | 1 cup | 48.3 |
| Peas, edible-podded, cooked | 1 cup | 40.0 |

| | | |
|---|---|---|
| Peas, green, canned, regular pk | 1 cup | 36.4 |
| Peas, green, frozen, | 1 cup | 38.4 |
| Pepper, green, raw | 1 cup | 1.0 |
| Peppers, sweet, green, cooked | 1 cup | 2.9 |
| Potato, baked | 1 | 4.0 |
| Potatoes, mashed, home-prepared whole milk & margarine added | 1 cup | 12.6 |
| Pumpkin, boiled, no salt | 1 cup | 2.0 |
| Pumpkin, canned, without salt | 1 cup | 39.2 |
| Sauerkraut, canned | 1 cup | 30.7 |
| Soybeans, cooked, boiled | 1 cup | 33.0 |
| Spinach, cooked | 1 cup | 1027.3 |
| Spinach, canned, drained solids | 1 cup | 987.8 |
| Spinach, raw leaf | 1 cup | 144.9 |
| Spring onion or scallion, raw | 1 cup | 207.0 |
| Swiss chard, raw | 1 cup | 299.0 |
| Tomato | 1 | 9.7 |
| Tomatoes, red, ripe, raw, | 1 cup | 14.2 |
| Tomato paste without salt | 1 cup | 29.9 |
| Turnip greens, boiled, drained | 1 cup | 29.3 |

| | | |
|---|---|---|
| Vegetables, mixed, frozen, cooked, boiled, drained, no salt | 1 cup | 29.1 |
| Vegetables, mixed, canned | 1 cup | 20.2 |
| Vegetable juice cocktail, canned | 1 cup | 12.8 |
| Watercress, raw | 1 cup | 85.0 |

## CONDIMENTS AND SWEETENERS

| | | |
|---|---|---|
| Gelatin | ½ cup | 0.0 |
| Honey | 1 tbsp | 0.0 |
| Peanut butter | 2 tbsp | 0.2 |
| Pickle, dill | 1 | 25.4 |
| Pickles, cucumber, dill | 1 | 11.9 |
| Salad dressing, French, regular | 1 tbsp | 18.9 |
| Salad dressing, vinegar and oil | 1 tbsp | 15.4 |
| Salad dressing, blue or Roquefort cheese dressing, regular | 1 tbsp | 13.9 |
| Salad dressing, Russian | 1 tbsp | 12.9 |
| Sugar, white, granulated | 1 tsp | 0.0 |
| Vegetable oil, canola | 1 tbsp | 17.1 |

## MISCELLANEOUS

| | | |
|---|---|---|
| Bread stuffing, bread, dry mix, prepared | 1/2 cup | 13.7 |
| Breakfast items, biscuit with egg and sausage | 1 | 14.4 |
| Candies, confectioner's coating, white | 1 cup | 13.9 |
| Eclairs, custard-filled with chocolate glaze | 1 | 17.5 |
| Seeds, pumpkin and squash seed kernels, roasted, w/salt added | 1 oz | 13.4 |
| Soup, vegetable, canned, chunky, ready-to-serve | 1 cup | 19.4 |
| Spices, parsley, dried | 1 tbsp | 17.7 |

Vitamin K is an important vitamin for other functions in your body so eliminating it all together would prevent its important role in bone development and bone maintenance.

# 22 QUESTIONS & ANSWERS

## Can I still drink coffee?

Coffee is one of the safest drinks we have and it is very good for you. It has more antioxidants than almost any food we consume. It should be safe for you to drink coffee while taking Warfarin, as long as you drink one or two cups per day consistently and monitor your INR levels.

## Is tea safe to drink?

While Black Tea leaves are high in Vitamin K when brewed there are very low amounts. It should be safe. Green tea and other types, as long as taken consistently, should be safe as well.

# I've read conflicting reports on cranberries and Warfarin. Should I avoid cranberries?

The *2003 United Kingdom's Committee on Safety of Medicines* alert to clinicians was probably the source of negative reactions to Warfarin resulting in even the medication's manufacturer recommending avoiding cranberries and cranberry juice. Two published studies have been conducted since then. In 2006 in the *Journal of the American Dietetic Association* and the other in 2009 in the *Journal of Clinical Pharmacology* reported no significant clinical interactions between Warfarin and drinking eight ounces of cranberry juice cocktail daily were found. Consequently, researchers concluded cranberry juice is safe to drink in small amounts while taking Warfarin, as long as your healthcare provider is aware that you are and your INR remains consistent.

# Do I have to give up alcohol?

Drinking alcohol does have an affect on how the liver metabolizes Warfarin. There is no need to stop consuming alcohol but a consistent daily intake should be limited to no more than one or two drinks. Excessive alcohol consumption can dangerously raise your INR.

# Where can I find more information?

The **Heart and Stroke Foundation**:

- Head office: Ottawa, Ontario (613) 569-4361

- Calgary, Alberta (403) 264 5549 or 1-888-473-4636

- Vancouver, British Columbia (604) 736-4404

- Winnipeg, Manitoba (204) 949-2000

- Saint John, New Brunswick (506) 634-1620 or

  1-800-663-3600

- Mount Pearl, Newfoundland (709) 753-8521

- Halifax, Nova Scotia (902) 423-7530 or

  1-800-423-4432

- Toronto, Ontario (416) 489-7111

- Charlottetown, Prince Edward Island (902) 892-7441

- Montreal, Quebec (514) 871-1551 or 1-800-567-8563

- Saskatoon, Saskatchewan (306) 244-2124

# Alphabetical Index

# ABOUT THE AUTHOR

Val Blake has been involved in the publishing industry for nearly 20 years. She authors and publishes international craft magazines, children's books, adult fiction, and non-fiction titles. She manages various websites and is an active contributor to online publications and many topical blogs.

CPSIA information can be obtained
at www.ICGtesting.com
Printed in the USA
LVOW04s2007180816
500950LV00010B/132/P